Cellulite Blaster

Quick Start Guide To Getting Rid Of Cellulite FAST and Blasting Them Off Your Stomach, Thighs, Legs & Butt!

by Aimee Blake
© Copyright 2017

(Health & Beauty Series - Book 4)

While all attempts have been made to verify the information provided in this publication, neither the author, nor the publisher assumes any responsibility for errors, omissions, or contrary interpretations on the subject matter herein. This book is for entertainment purposes only. The views expressed are those of the author alone, and should not be taken as expert instruction or commands.

The reader is responsible for his or her own actions. A few affiliate links are included throughout this book. All products recommended have been personally used and tested by the author. Reader or purchaser are advised to do their own research before making any purchase online.

Adherence to all applicable laws and regulations, including international, federal, state, and local governing professional licensing, business practices, advertising, and all other aspects of doing business in the US, Canada, Australia or any other jurisdiction is the sole responsibility of the reader or purchaser.

Neither the author nor the publisher assumes any responsibility or liability whatsoever on the behalf of the purchaser or reader of these materials. Any perceived slight of any individual or organization is purely unintentional.

Table of Contents

Chapter 1: What Causes Cellulite

Cellulite has long been associated with negative processes such as aging and weight gain. It is no surprise then that many people are looking to boost their body confidence by reducing the appearance of "orange peel" skin and "dimpling."

Before discussing the various methods that claim to be a cure, let's first examine the internal physiological factors that **cause** cellulite. We will also look at the lifestyle factors that you can change in order to improve the quality of the skin.

Anatomy of the skin and cellulite

The skin is the largest organ in the body and has multiple functions. These include our sense of touch, our ability to maintain a constant temperature, and our ability to fight off infections and foreign bodies.

The skin is made up of three layers:
- Epidermis
- Dermis
- and Subcutaneous tissue.

Other structures of the integumentary system include hair follicles, sweat glands, and pores, all of which can impact on the appearance of the skin.

The epidermis is the outermost layer of the skin and is essentially a barrier between the body and the outside world. This is also the layer with the highest rate of cell removal and renewal.

Underneath the epidermis lies the dermis. The dermis is principally involved in perception, defense, and thermoregulation.

The structure of the dermis includes bundles of collagen proteins interspersed with elastin fibers. These give the skin its firmness and elasticity.

Finally, the subcutaneous tissue is a fatty layer below the dermis. These layer stores lipids, and protects and insulates the body. It is this layer of fat, rather than deeper adipose tissue, that contributes to the appearance of cellulite.

Why does cellulite form?

Cellulite is primarily a result of fat redistribution within the body, with dimples and lumps most frequently forming around the thighs and buttocks.

Studies have found that a weakening of the capillary walls, **fascia in distress** can cause plasma (fluid) to move into the surrounding adipose (fat) tissue.

These adipose cells then clump together and bend the supporting collagen fibers, connecting tissue, causing undesirable lumps and bumps.

What most people don't tell you is fascia that is distress will adhere to your skin and cause visible dimples. "Fascia adhesions can pull the skin down and force the fat up, causing dents and dimples commonly known as cellulite

This process has a snowball effect wherein the accumulation of cellulite cells leads to poorer circulation, which results in even more cellulite.

Cellulite can be graded into four categories, depending on the appearance of the skin and structure of the cells.

Grade 1 implies that while there are underlying changes to the adipose cells, there is no visual evidence of cellulite.

At Grade 2 cellulite may be exposed if the skin is pinched, but is still essentially invisible. The skin may be pasty and cool as a result of decreased circulation.

At Grade 3 cellulite becomes more obvious. Rough "orange peel" skin is visible on standing.

Grade 4 cellulite is visible on lying and standing and includes all the symptoms of the first three grades.

Factors affecting the formation of cellulite

The causes of cellulite are multifaceted and factors such as genetics, circulation, activity levels, and gender all have a much larger role to play than weight or age.

Although losing weight may reduce the appearance of dimpled skin, women of all sizes can develop cellulite. Skin becomes thinner with age which can make cellulite more visible, but age itself is not an underlying cause.

There may be injuries to your body, illnesses that cause internal scar tissue like adhesions which damages your fascia (connective tissue) and stops blood from flowing to the area.

Due to the impact of blood vessel structure on the formation of cellulite, areas that receive low levels of blood flow are more likely to develop an orange peel appearance. Therefore, sedentary lifestyles may lead to higher levels of cellulite.

The lack of blood, circulation and distressed fascia are one of the main reasons of the formation of cellulite.

Cellulite is also more commonly found in women due to the anatomical layout of the septae which attach the skin to the fat. These septae lie straight in females which results in visible dimpling.

In men, these septae lie at an angle which disguises the formation of cellulite. Laxity of these structures over time will also contribute to the appearance of subcutaneous fat.

The majority of women will develop cellulite at some point in life, regardless of weight or body shape.

Lifestyle factors, such as smoking, also impact on cellulite formation. Smoking has many detrimental effects on the body. Cigarette smoking leads to the destruction of cells, including blood vessels. It also poorly affects the circulatory system by slowing blood flow, all of which increase the causative factors of cellulite.

Chapter 2: Cellulite Myths

There are so many myths surrounding cellulite. If we were to believe everything we hear about the causes and cures of cellulite, we could waste a ridiculous amount of time and money trying things that never had a chance of working.

In this chapter we will discuss four of the most common myths surrounding cellulite formation and treatment, and the reasons why they are simply not true.

Myth 1: Cellulite is big chunks of excess fat and only overweight people get it

One of the most persistent myths about cellulite is that its big chunks of fat and only overweight people can get it.

This belief comes from the incorrect assumption that areas of cellulite are just chunks of excess fat that have accumulated in the body, and that losing weight will magically remove them.

Unfortunately, 95% of women will develop cellulite, regardless of body weight. All humans have fat (albeit some more than others) and we can all be susceptible to the poor circulation and lax collagen fibers that lead to cellulite.

What healthy weight loss will do is reduce the visibility of "cottage cheese" skin but it does not get rid of it.

It's not fat, it's Fascia!

In Ashley black's the "Cellulite Myth" book - she states that fat is not the problem. There is absolutely NO chemical difference between the fat cells in areas of cellulite and the fat in any other area of the body.

In fact, the appearance of cellulite is not about fat at all, it's about connective tissue called **fascia**. First, you need to know that we literally have fascia in every nook and cranny of our bodies and it's all connected like a giant sticky web.

Fascia is the connective tissue that holds everything inside us in place. It's the reason your ribs don't poke through your skin and your liver isn't falling into your stomach and crushing it.

Your cellulite is caused by unhealthy fascia that creates fascial adhesions and distortions to your body NOT big chunks of fat.

Myth 2: Cellulite is caused by toxins in the body

In spite of the claims of many creams and cures, toxins are not the cause of cellulite. Poor circulation, collagen damage, and changes to cell structure are.

Detoxing has a number of benefits, including brighter skin, but it won't do a thing to treat your cellulite. Many products, magazines, and websites claim that certain foods or juices or products will remove the cellulite-causing toxins, but be wary of such assertions because there is little evidence to back them up.

Myth 3: Cellulite is an inevitable fact of aging /genetics / womanhood

This myth has a basis in truth. Many people do develop cellulite because of heredity or gender or increasing age. This is particularly true for post-menopausal women as the drop in estrogen leads to a weakening of blood vessels and connective tissue.

But that does not mean that we cannot prevent cellulite formation or improve the appearance of existing cellulite.
It is also important to remember that anyone can get cellulite. There are men and young people who have cellulite.

So the idea that cellulite is an issue only for older women is completely false.

Myth 4: The cure for cellulite is extreme weight loss / tanning / special clothing

Weight loss may reduce the appearance of cellulite to a certain extent, but extreme weight loss over a short period of time will almost certainly make it worse.

Losing large amounts of weight very quickly leaves you liable to weak and sagging skin, which can present as skin folds, stretch marks, and very visible cellulite. You are better served by a regime of regular exercise and a high quality nutritious diet.

Tanned skin, via sun bed or fake tan, can make the body visually slimmer and reduce the appearance of cellulite. However, claims that UV rays from the sun or from sun beds will cure cellulite are completely unfounded.

Tanning without sunscreen also puts you at higher risk for skin damage, sunburn, and melanoma.

While special "cellulite curing" clothing may reduce the appearance of cellulite while you are wearing it, there is no evidence to suggest that this improves the quality of the skin or has any lasting effect.

It may even cut off circulation to certain areas of the body, making cellulite worse. Don't lose money by getting sucked into claims that cannot be backed up.

The closest form of CURE for cellulite is...

- Breaking up the fascial adhesions that are clamping down on the tissues and restoring the fascia to get smooth, healthy skin.

- **Followed** with a healthy clean diet and plenty of hydration to give your body the best chance of healing itself through vitamins and nutrition.

Chapter 3: Cellulite Blasting

Lately, there's been a growing trend of women who are "blasting" their cellulite and loose skin with a stick called the "FasciaBlaster" *(I'm one of them).*

I wrote this book before I knew about the "FasciaBlaster" and in this updated version of Cellulite Blaster, it deserves it's own chapter in this book.

Who created the FasciaBlaster?

Ashley Black is a fitness instructor, massage therapist and the creator of the FasciaBlaster. She created the FasciaBlaster because of her history of Juvenile Rheumatoid Arthritis and spent years from suffering severe bouts of pain.

What is Fascia?

Fascia is the fibrous connective tissue that runs throughout our body, fused to every vein and artery, bone and muscle. The 'myofascial' system is the medical term for the 'fascia tissue' tightly connecting our body's insides.

Because it weaves through nerves, fat, and muscle it can inadvertently render negative effects. Due to poor diet, strenuous physical activity, non-ergonomic practices, and genetics.

The negative effects can consist of cellulite, arthritis, joint conditions, muscle under development, neck and back pain, nerve reaction, just to name a few..

What is the FasciaBlaster?

The FasciaBlaster was originally by created by Ashley Black for the purpose of loosening and reorganizing the fascia around joints, giving one's relief from arthritis, adhesion, and pain.

The Fascia Blaster has been proven to reduce and eliminate joint pain. It also has become popular for its positive effects on the appearance of cellulite.

It has become acknowledged by doctors, therapists (including massage therapists), sports figures and trainers for eliminating pain (including nerve, muscle and joint pain), stiffness, bad circulation, and reduced the look of cellulite based on real results from real people.

The results I have experienced along with other women have been amazing. Although my cellulite has not disappeared entirely, it has DEFINITELY diminished.

Her Facebook group is at Facebook.com/groups/FasciaBlasters/. Just hit the request button to join the group, it's free to join and you can see everyone's progress photos before you decide to buy the Fascia Blaster.

I receive no remuneration for recommending the FasciaBlaster in this book. I just want to share with you that it

WORKS and has become a staple in my weekly routine to stave off cellulite as well as adhesions in my back due to a car accident I had when I was 16.

How do you use the FasciaBlaster?
The FasciaBlaster works by breaking up and softening the fascia tissue that bonds our body together like glue.

By realigning the fascia and allowing fluids and fats to be released and flow correctly the fascia is able to become re-hydrated, thus maximizing the full potential of healthy fascia and eliminating trapped fat.

In addition regulating nerves and blood flow, enables muscle growth where it once was impeded by constricting tight and/or knotted fascia.

As you can see in the picture above, the claws have smooth round balls at the end, which act as super powerful fingers per-se.

By massaging the body with the FasciaBlaster following the recommended technique along with plenty of Oil ~ will encourage highly positive results!

It looks like a pretty simple tool, however the science behind it is the magic at work. There are other types of devices that claim similar results; however the FasciaBlaster is the only tool on the market that breaks up fascia and delivers such highly proven results consistently!

Routine for Cellulite Fascia Blasting:

Step 1: Warm up internally with 15minutes of low impact cardio and warm up externally with a hot shower, bath, sauna or heating pads. Fascia loves heat because it increases circulation and puts the fascia in a pliable state.

Step 2: Take your clothes off and apply coconut oil. The FasciaBlaster works on bare skin, apply coconut oil on your thighs, stomach or any trouble areas.

Step 3: Get your fascia blasting stick and start blasting by rubbing the stick onto your skin. Gently glide the blaster up and down, side to side in every direction - just not in circles.

How hard should you blast?

I'll leave it to Ashley to explain it in this video here: Youtube.com/watch?v=Ro5PLVOLpsM

Chapter 4: Cellulite Diet

Simply losing weight will do nothing to reduce the appearance of cellulite. As we have already established, cellulite plagues fat and thin individuals alike.

But can the quality of the food we eat contribute to the development of cottage cheese skin?

The main aims in the battle against cellulite are to reduce water retention and strengthen the collagen fibers that prevent the adipose cells from clumping together.

This means increasing your intake of Vitamin C, polyunsaturated fats, lean protein, and fiber, while cutting out foods that cause you to retain fluid.

Foods to fight cellulite

Vitamin C: While all vitamins are beneficial to the skin, Vitamin C in particular has properties which strengthen the collagen in the dermis.

It is also involved in skin healing and is a top food for reducing cellulite. Instead of relying on vitamins, try to icrease your Vitamin C intake with oranges, strawberries, tomatoes, broccoli, and bell peppers.

Many of these same foods contain bioflavanoids, which both improve circulation and correct imbalances in the cells. Garlic, spinach, and citrus fruits are great sources of this super-vitamin.

Polyunsaturated fats: These are the "good" fats. The main role of polyunsaturated fats is to reduce the amount of low-density cholesterol in the blood stream (this is the cholesterol that contributes to cardiovascular disease).

Healthy circulation is a key part of fighting cellulite. These fats will also aid hydration in the skin. Polyunsaturated fats include Omega-3 and Omega-6 fatty acids which can be found in mackerel, salmon, and nuts. These good fats can also be found in flax seed, linseed, and olive oil.

Fiber: Fiber falls under the category of carbohydrates and is a structural component in plants and crops. Although it is found in many of our foods, it is actually indigestible by the human body.

Because of this, high fiber foods are low calorie, filling, and promote regular bowel motions and excretion of excess fluid. If you want to avoid bloating, fill up on fiber.

Good sources of fiber include apples, bran, whole grain breads and cereals, and lentils.

Antioxidants: Although detoxing isn't the solution to cellulite, antioxidant rich food is fantastic for fighting fluid retention due to their hydrating and nutrient rich qualities.

Drink green tea throughout the day, and enhance your meals with cayenne pepper and turmeric.

Berries can act as the perfect snack or a dessert. One specific antioxidant, lycopene, is known to stimulate circulation and can be found in tomatoes and apricots.

Natural diuretics: Some foods just flush the excess water out of your body, relieving your skin of excess fluid. Include cucumber and celery to a salad or sandwich, and have a glass of cranberry juice on the side.

Foods to avoid

Salt: Other than reducing the amount of salt you add to food, start to develop an awareness of the amount of salt that is hidden in your food.

Processed foods, particularly fried foods and fast foods, contain an enormous amount of salt (salt is a readily available preservative), so your intake could be higher than you realize.

Control the amount of salt in your food by preparing and cooking your own meals whenever possible. Stick to the guideline of 6g a day for an adult.

Sugar: While there is naturally occurring fructose in many fruits and vegetables, the amount of processed sugar that is present in modern day foods is phenomenal.

And don't think that this only refers to candy and ice cream; refined carbohydrates such as white bread, pastries, and pasta also contain high levels of sugar.

Water retention and bloating are common side effects of a highly refined sugary diet. Sugar will also cause adipose tissue to swell, making cellulite more visible.

Alcohol: Small amounts of alcohol cause no real problem. Larger amounts of alcohol, particularly if taken in one sitting, can do detrimental damage to the cells of the body.

Drinking also lends itself to bloating, dehydration, and fluid retention, all of which are key contributing factors to the formation of cellulite.

If you add sugar-filled mixers into the equation, you are seriously decreasing your ability to fight cellulite. If you choose to drink, be sure to keep within the recommended allowance of alcohol units for your age, gender, and body weight.

Nicotine: Nicotine isn't a food but it is something that is taken into the body and damages the cells. When attempting to reduce cellulite, it is essential to build up the body's internal structures, not break them down further.

Smoking increases the appearance of aging, makes ligaments and collagen fibers more lax, and dehydrates the skin. To get rid of cellulite, you have to get rid of the cigarettes.

Chapter 5: Cellulite Exercises

Regular exercise increases strength, maintains cardiovascular health, and releases endorphins (those chemicals in the brain that put us in a good mood).

Exercise also offers specific benefits to the reduction of cellulite. By working the areas that are affected by cellulite, we can increase muscle tone, strengthen connective tissue, stimulate lymphatic drainage, and boost circulation.

You can also reduce the size of adipose cells (which will make cellulite less visible) by doing regular cardiovascular activity. Such activities can be used as a warm up for your strength exercises, and also as a workout all on their own.

Fitting three thirty minute cardio sessions into your week can do wonders for your physical and mental health. Choose from a wide range of sports and activities, such as walking, running, swimming, cycling, dancing, or team sports.

NOTE - However be careful not to overdo it with exercise especially if you already have existing injuries. Old injuries carry scar tissue and adhesion which restricts blood flows and damages your fascia.

If you already have pain, it may be caused from damaged fascia and a lack of blood flow to the area. If this is the case, stick to light exercise and blast your body with the "FasciaBlaster".

Exercises to fight cellulite

The exercises below are designed to target the most common problem areas for the cellulite – butt, hips, and thighs.

To complete the following exercises, you will need an exercise mat, a chair (or barre), and (optional) hand weights.

Complete 2-3 sets of 10-15 reps, depending on your strength and fitness level.

The first five exercises are performed standing, while the last five are performed on the floor.

Wall squat

1. Stand with your back against a wall with your feet pointing forward. Bring your feet about a foot in front of you.
2. Slide your back down the wall into a squat position.
3. Hold for 20 – 60 seconds.

Barre raise

1. Place your hands on the back of a steady chair (or barre). Stand up straight and tall.
2. With your heel pointed towards the ceiling, raise your right foot behind you.

3. Bring your leg as high as you can while maintaining good form.
4. Repeat on the left side.

Romanian dead lift

1. Stand up straight, toes pointed forwards, and knees slightly bent.
2. If you are using weights, hold one in each hand with your arms in front of your thighs.
3. Keeping your back straight, lead with the weights and bend at the hips, bringing the weights towards the floor as you inhale.
4. Exhale as you return to your starting position.

Reverse lunge

1. Starting with feet together, bring your right foot about a foot behind you.
2. Inhale as you lunge straight down.
3. Do not let your knee go over the toes. If this happens, you need a wider stance.
4. Exhale as you return to the starting position.
5. Repeat on the opposite side and continue to alternate.

Side step
1. With your hands clasped in front of your chest, stand with your feet wider than hips width apart.
2. Bring all your weight to your right foot, using the left only for balance.

3. With a quick hop, change positions so that your weight is now in your left foot.

4. Jump between the two positions for the appropriate number of repetitions.

Sitting kick

1. From a sitting position, bring both legs straight in front of you. Keep your back straight and bend your left knee so that your left foot is on the floor.

2. Keeping your right leg straight, lift your right foot up towards the ceiling as you exhale.

3. Inhale as you return to the starting position.

4. Repeat the exercise on the opposite side.

Bridge

1. Lie on your back with both knees bent up and feet on the floor. Rest your arms along your sides for support.
2. As you exhale, lift the hips up towards the ceiling.
3. Return to the starting position as you inhale.

Inner thigh lift

1. Lie on your right side. Keep your body in a straight line, parallel with the mat, and rest your head on your upper arm.
2. Bring your left arm in front of you for light support.
3. Bend your top leg, placing the foot in front of your bottom knee. Keeping

the bottom leg straight, lift it up as you exhale.

4. Inhale as you lower the bottom leg down.
5. Repeat exercise on the other side.

Donkey kick

1. Start on all fours with your knees directly below your hips and your wrists below your shoulders.
2. Keeping the bend in your knee, bring your right leg straight up, as if you wanted to kick the ceiling.
3. Return to starting the position
4. repeat on the opposite side.

Fire hydrant

Start on all fours with your knees directly below your hips and your wrists below your shoulders.

Keeping the bend in your knee, lift your right leg to the side (like a dog peeing on a fire hydrant). Return to the starting position and repeat on the opposite side.

Chapter 6: At Home Cellulite Treatments

Before you bring in the professionals, there is a whole host of at-home options that can be used to treat cellulite.

These range from DIY recipes and massage techniques to home versions of the devices used by beauticians and dermatologists.

In this chapter, we will wade through the benefits of these home treatments, expose any false claims, explore the pros and cons of each, and give you a few free (or very cheap) options to try along the way.

Body brushing

Dry brushing has been shown to improve circulation, exfoliate the skin, and stimulate the lymphatic system.

Increased blood flow to problem areas will bathe the cells in oxygen and nutrients, making adipose cells less likely to clump together and collagen fibers stronger and less likely to buckle.

Better lymphatic function will lead to more efficient drainage of excess fluid from the body, which both prevents and improves cellulite.

Dry brushing should be carried out before a shower or bath, using a brush with stiff, natural fibers. At first, two to three sessions a week should be sufficient, but you can do this more frequently if you wish.

- Prepare your skin by rubbing coconut oil into problem areas *(this step is optional but has been shown to improve results.)*
- Brush firmly along the skin, starting at the feet, and working your way up the body in the direction of the heart.
- If you choose to brush your abdomen, make circular strokes from the back around to the navel.
- Avoid sensitive areas such as the breasts, genitals, face, and underarms when dry brushing.
- Rinse the skin with warm water to remove dead skin cells. Afterwards, moisturize deeply.

- I use this dry brush at Amzn.to/ 2fU7bvk.

Fascia Blasting

As mentioned in Chapter 3, I use the FasciaBlaster tool created by Ashley black. In fact, I dry brush first before I shower then once I'm in the shower, I start fascia blasting.

Routine for Fascia Blasting:

Step 1: Warm up internally with 15minutes of low impact cardio and warm up externally with a hot shower, bath, sauna or heating pads. Fascia loves heat because it increases circulation and puts the fascia in a pliable state.

Step 2: Take your clothes off and apply coconut oil. The FasciaBlaster works on bare skin, apply coconut oil on your thighs, stomach or any trouble areas.

Step 3: Get your fascia blasting stick and start blasting by rubbing the stick onto your skin. Gently glide the blaster up and down, side to side in every direction - just not in circles.

How hard should you blast?

I'll leave it to Ashley to explain it in this video here: Youtube.com/watch?v=Ro5PLVOLpsM

DIY slimming wraps

Slimming wraps utilize compression and body heat to reduce cellulite by clearing out toxins and excess fluid.

This treatment requires time and preparation but is favored by many (including a number of celebrities) as a quick, short-term solution to stubborn cellulite.

No matter what recipe you use, you will need ace bandages (or strips of cloth), Saran wrap, and lots of water (to stay hydrated!)

The recipe below is for a basic wrap. You can then customize this recipe to suit your needs.

Basic wrap recipe

- Boil two liters of water.
- Ingredients should be added to boiling water and then left to cool for ten to fifteen minutes before applying to the skin.
- Add a cup of salt, which will draw toxins and fluid out of the body via osmosis.
- Add a few drops of essential oils to moisturize the skin.

Alternative liquids: Add green tea bags to your boiling water to boost the antioxidant properties of your slimming wrap.

Replace a cup of water with a cup of lemon juice to cleanse the skin cells with citric acid. If you have dry and itchy skin, replace a cup of water with a cup of full fat milk.

Salts: Epsom salts are the most commonly used salts in slimming wraps, but any sea salt will have detoxifying properties.

Clays: Clays will exfoliate and detoxify the skin while boosting circulation. Add 2 cups of green clay for oily skin, or red clay for dry skin. Check that your chosen clay is compatible with your skin type.

Essential oils: Add a few drops of your chosen oil to boost the benefits of your skin wrap. Rosehip oil works wonders on a number of skin blemishes.

Tea tree and Aloe Vera are well known for their gentle healing properties. Olive oil is filled with Vitamin E, while Shea oil promotes skin elasticity.

Using the body wrap

1. Soak the ace bandages in your mixture.
2. Warm your mixture to open up the pores and to make for a more pleasant experience.
3. Wrap the ace bandages around the area. Make sure that the bandages are tight, but not so tight that it will cut off your circulation.
4. Cover the ace bandages in Saran wrap to retain moisture.
5. Cover yourself in a washable blanket to keep warm and relax for

at least sixty minutes before washing off.

6. Ensure you stay hydrated by sipping on water.

DIY cellulite scrubs

Homemade scrubs reduce cellulite physically, by stimulating the blood vessels of the skin (through exfoliation and mild abrasion), and chemically, through the properties of its additives.

The recipe below is a basic sugar scrub. However, there is a section on "additives" which are ingredients you can add to your scrub. Caffeine, for example, is a natural antioxidant and vasodilator, which reduces toxins and increases blood flow.

Make sure to store scrubs in a sealed, plastic container in a cool environment. Use within seven days.

Basic scrub recipe

- Choose a carrier oil for your scrub, such as almond or jojoba.
- Olive oil and vegetable oil are also perfect options, as is simple baby oil.
- Choose an abrasive. Any salt or sugar with small granules can be used. Brown sugar is gentler to sensitive skin.
- Add one part oil to two parts abrasive e.g. ½ cup brown sugar to ¼ cup jojoba oil.
- Add your preferred additive.

- Mix well before use, as contents will settle.

Additives to scrubs

Caffeine: Reduce the amount of abrasive you use by one-third and replace it with ground coffee e.g. ½ cup oil to 1/3 cup coffee grounds and 2/3 cup sugar.

Cayenne pepper: Add a teaspoon of cayenne to your scrub to heat up the skin and boost blood flow and metabolism.

Juniper oil: Add a few drops of juniper oil to your scrub to gain the diuretic, anti-rheumatic benefits of this stimulant. This recipe can also be turned into an effective massage oil by leaving out the abrasive.

Massage techniques

Massage works on a similar principle to dry brushing. Pressure on the cells boosts circulation and lymphatic function, which prevents and reduces cellulite.

Massage techniques can be performed on dry skin, but is more optimally carried out with essential oils like Avocado oil, coconut oil or sweet almond oil.

Massage has the added benefits of relieving muscle tension and promoting relaxation.

- Using a lotion, cream, or oil, make firm, circular motions along the area with the tips of the fingers.
- Use as much pressure as you are comfortable with, always moving in the direction of the heart.
- Start to lift and pinch small areas of the skin in a kneading fashion.
- Next, lift and pinch large areas of the skin and gently twist, as if you were wringing water from a towel.
- Use your knuckles to apply firm pressure along the area.
- Start by applying stationary pressure and releasing.
- Work up to making circular motions along your body with your knuckles.
- Always move in the direction of your heart.

Over the counter cellulite creams

Over the counter cellulite creams come with a wide range of claims, costs, and convenience. When you are shopping for a cellulite cream, know that no cream will magically remove your cellulite.

Good creams will have cosmeceutical ingredients that will reduce the appearance of cellulite with regular use but they are NOT a permanent solution.

When deciding whether or not to try a cream, it is important to ask how much time commitment this treatment requires, that the ingredients are NOT toxic and whether it really works at all.

There are obvious benefits of course. Although prices of these creams vary, they are unlikely to break the bank. Most of the cellulite creams have few side effects although there is the possible risk of allergic reaction.

Cellulite creams are designed to smooth and plump up the skin. Often times, they contain caffeine and other circulation boosting ingredients, as well as retinol A and antioxidants.

The following creams are five of the most popular on the market. Below is a summary of how they work, what they actually do, and the price you can expect to pay for each.

Revitol Cellulite Solution

What it does: This easy to apply cream claims to reduce the appearance of dimples with all natural ingredients. The key ingredients in Revitol are Retinol A and caffeine, which increase blood flow to hard to reach areas and tighten the skin.

Effectiveness: Revitol is a leader in the cosmetics industry and their Cellulite Solution is frequently found in best buy lists for anti-cellulite creams.

Although it has not been clinically tested, in a number of consumer tests users found it reduced the appearance of cellulite after four weeks. To see improvements, it is necessary to apply the cream three to four times a day.

Price or Revitol: $40

Where to buy Revitol: Amzn.to/
2vRsMIC

Celluvin

What it does: The makers of Celluvin claim that this cream will reduce cellulite, replenish moisture, and give an overall more youthful appearance to the skin.

As well as containing caffeine and retinol A, Celluvin includes rosehip seed oil, glycerin, vitamin E, and collagen on its ingredients list.

Effectiveness: Celluvin has rated highly in clinical research and tests, as well as being extremely well received by consumers. Due to its potent mix of skin nourishing ingredients, Celluvin has been proven to detoxify and moisturize the skin, renew skin cells, improve circulation, and strengthen the skin's elasticity in order to reduce the appearance of cellulite.

This product requires application twice a day to see results. As an added perk, Celluvin comes with free delivery and a ninety-day money back guarantee.

Price of Celluvin: $54.95

Where to buy Celluvin: Amzn.to/ 2x06tRe

Fat Girl Slim

What it does: This cream, by Bliss, claims to improve lymphatic drainage, boost circulation, and reduce the appearance of dimpled skin.

Caffeine molecules contained within a fast acting cream are designed to quickly reduce any signs of cellulite. The cream is available as a stand alone item, or as part of Bliss' cellulite banishing bundles.

Effectiveness: Although Fat Girl Slim comes with the esthetician seal of approval, this brand's experience and fame may outweigh the cream's actual effectiveness.

While customer reviews are good, there is no clinical testing to back this up. This cream requires application twice a day for best results.

Price of Fat Girl Slim: $30

Where to buy Fat Girl Slim: Amzn.to/2vRBF50

Cellulean

What it does: Cellulean is designed to firm the skin and improve skin elasticity to decrease cellulite in as little as two weeks. It also contains aminophylline which is thought to decrease the size of adipose cells. The product also comes with a free thirty-day trial.

Effectiveness: Although the product claims to use pharmaceutical grade ingredients, no concise ingredient list is provided, so personal research on the product proves difficult.

Noted ingredients include caffeine, salicylic acid, and aminophylline, although no details are provided as to how these ingredients interact with each other.

However, the Cellulean website does contain details of nine reputable clinical studies which back up the cream's claims. Cellulean requires daily application for optimal results.

Price of Cellulean: $79.95

Where to buy Cellulean:

Amzn.to/2fTPs77 (Amazon has it discounted to $32)

Murad Firm and Tone Serum

What it does: From one of the leading companies in skincare and product development comes Firm and Tone Serum, which offers improved circulation, heightened skin elasticity, and targeted cellulite treatment.

The ingredients in the serum – including cayenne pepper and caffeine – are delivered down into the skin by liposomes which ensure that the effects of the cream reach even the deepest areas.

Effectiveness: Independent clinical trials attest to Murad's claims but customer reviews are mixed. The serum appears to be quite effective on a short term basis but does not offer the same lasting effects as similarly priced products.

Murad Firm and Tone Serum comes with a sixty-day money back guarantee and the company offers excellent support and an easy returns policy.

Price of Murad Firm and Tone: $75

Where to buy Murad Firm and Tone: Amzn.to/2uRnIH2 (Amazon has it discounted to $43)

At home devices

There are now many at home equivalents to the cellulite treating devices used by professionals.

While these devices are significantly more expensive than creams and serums, they can be seen as an investment item which can save you money in the long run.

We look at three of the most popular types of at-home devices and give you the information to decide whether these devices are worth the splurge.

Ultrasonic cavitation

What it does: Ultrasonic cavitation works by destroying adipose cells in localized areas with ultrasound waves.

The cell remnants are then metabolized by the body and later excreted.

This method can be used to shape and sculpt the body, as well as enhancing overall fat loss. This non-invasive pain-free treatment can be used twice a week and boasts few side effects (besides possible temporary skin redness).

Many machines come with a radio frequency function in order to combine this method and the method below.

Effectiveness: Reviews are mixed. While some users claim that these at-home devices work wonders, most doctors will remind you that devices must be extremely low powered in order to be used without medical supervision.

Machines appear to have a positive effect over time, but don't expect the same results that you would see from a professional.

Popular products:
CaviSculpt Home Ultrasound Cavitation Lipo
Home Cavitation Slimming System (Cavi EVO+)
Cost: $575 - $2000

Where to buy:
Amzn.to/2x03ats

Tripolar radio frequency
What it does: Tripolar radio frequency is used to tighten and strengthen collagen fibers. By heating the dermal and epidermal layers of the skin, these

fibers are forced to contract and the stimulation of the skin triggers heightened metabolism.

Over time this causes synthesis of new collagen fibers and thickening of the dermal layer, resulting in smoother, lifted skin. Many machines come with an ultrasonic cavitation function in order to achieve maximum effectiveness.

Effectiveness: Reviews from dermatologists and users alike are slightly more positive for radio frequency. Although it is still a lower strength version of the radio frequency used by the pros, it does appear to reduce the appearance of cellulite (as well as wrinkles and other blemishes) over time.

Popular products:
Tripollar Apollo
High Frequency D'arsonval Home Use Device
Cost: $300 - $500

Where to buy:
Amzn.to/2wbh7H8

Lipomassage
What it does: Lipomassage is a non-invasive method of cellulite reduction which utilizes motorized rollers and valves to contour the body and tighten the skin.

These rollers target stubborn fat cells and burn them through vigorous stimulation. The treatment is also used to encourage circulation and relieve muscle pain.

Effectiveness: Lipomassage is approved by the FDA for the treatment of cellulite. The treatment appears to provide excellent temporary effects, but these only seem to as long as the treatment is being carried out.

More significant results may be found in attending Endermologie appointments with trained professionals.

Popular products:
Wellbox Self Lipomassage
Lipomassage by Endermologie
Cost: $900 - $1600

Chapter 7: Cosmetic Cellulite Treatment

Unfortunately, some cellulite just won't disappear in spite of your best efforts. If persistent cellulite is getting you down, you may need to consult with a professional.

A variety of professions deal with cellulite removal, including estheticians, dermatologists, and plastic surgeons. A number of effective treatments have been developed in recent years, such as carboxytherapy, mesotherapy, and ultra-cavitation and radio frequency **however they do have side effects.**

Although advances in technology have grown in leaps and bounds, I don't recommend going under the knife just to get rid of cellulite. <u>The risk of infection, adhesion, damage to fascia and scar tissue is high.</u>

Sometimes, it's a matter of sticking to a routine and method for 3 months before you can actually see any results. Just remember to take before and after so that you can truly see if it's working or not.

With that said, let's explore the current cosmetic treatments available for cellulite.

Ultrasonic cavitation and radio frequency multipolar

How it works: This non-surgical, non-invasive treatment professionally combines the techniques of the home devices described in the previous chapter.

Ultrasonic cavitation uses ultrasound waves to penetrate deep into the skin and cause fat cell membranes to break down and liquidize. The body then discharges the fat via the excretory and lymphatic systems.

Multipolar radio frequency treatments have different roles in tackling cellulite. Monopolar radio frequency uses heat to emulsify triglycerides and adipose cells so that they can be more easily metabolized by the body.

Tripolar radio frequency speeds the expulsion of the liquidized adipose tissue from the area and causes the collagen fibers surrounding them to contract. This results in tighter, lifted skin, and increased collagen and elastin synthesis.

Pros: Because it is non-invasive, ultrasonic cavitation and radio frequency does not require surgery, anesthetic nor recovery time, and the procedure only takes forty to sixty minutes.

It is advisable to stay hydrated and reduce stimulants such as caffeine and alcohol before and after the treatment.

This would be the first cosmetic treatment option I would recommend.

Cons: Some people may experience nausea or skin redness after the treatment, but this is short lasting.

It is unsuitable for those who are pregnant or have a pacemaker, heart disease, or kidney disease.

It can also take ten to twelve sessions to see substantial results, and each session could cost anywhere from $150 to $300 per area.

Carboxytherapy

How it works: Carboxytherapy refers to the subcutaneous injection of carbon dioxide into the area affected by cellulite.

Working on the principle of "oxygen off-loading," the added carbon dioxide triggers a boost in circulation so that the red blood cells can carry the carbon dioxide back to the lungs for exhalation.

This leads to increased oxygen flow to the area. It is also thought to stimulate collagen production and improve skin elasticity. Specific injection techniques can also burst the fatty deposits which contribute to cellulite.

Pros: Reviews of carboxytherapy are resoundingly positive. No down time is required post-treatment, and no pain should be experienced during the procedure.

Each session lasts only fifteen to thirty minutes, so it is a quick and convenient option. **It's also been used to treat dark under eye circles and stretch marks.**

No foreign substances are being introduced into the body, as it is naturally equipped to excrete carbon dioxide.

Cons: Bruising at the injection site is a common complaint, particularly when the lower body is being treated. It may take ten to twenty sessions to see results.

Whilst non-invasive, carboxytherapy does involve injections, so keep this in mind if you are needle-phobic.

The treatment costs $400 to $1000. It has not been clinically tested by the FDA.

Mesotherapy
How it works: Originating in France, mesotherapy treats cellulite by administering micro-injections into the mesodermal layer of the skin (the small area between the epidermis and the dermis.)

These injections can contain vitamins, homeopathic remedies, plant extracts, or prescribed medication. These chemicals are designed to break down adipose cells, which will then be metabolized by the body.

Pros: Users who had a positive experience with a reputable doctor have revealed amazing results from mesotherapy, so it is worth doing your research to find an experienced and qualified practitioner. Sessions are only forty five minutes long.

Cons: Side effects include bruising, risk of infection, and unevenness with a lumpy effect as the liquid that is injected burns the fat cell but doesn't necessarily spread evenly underneath the skin. The procedure is not approved by the FDA and many doctors are wary of using these injections.

The cost of mesotherapy varies hugely, but can be up to $2,500.

Cellulaze

How it works: Cellulaze is a procedure carried out by a surgeon and involves making small incisions at the site of the cellulite and inserting a laser fiber into the skin.

The laser will be guided through a cannula which will release the fibers that tug at the skin and break down offending fat cells in order to smooth out the surface. Cellulaze also thickens the dermal layer of the skin and promotes collagen production.

Pros: Cellulaze only requires one session to treat cellulite, and is FDA approved. The overwhelming majority of women who have undergone the procedure have found it effective in reducing the appearance of cellulite. The results of Cellulaze are permanent.

Cons: Soreness and bruising are common side effects, and recovery time can vary from person to person. Since it requires surgery, the risk of infection, bacteria can occur and some women have reported adhesion and lumpiness resulting in bumpy contours.

You will also be required to wear compression stockings for a period after the procedure in order to prevent clotting. Cellulaze can cost up to $7000, and it takes three to six months to see results.

Liposuction

How it works: Liposuction removes unwanted deposits of fat by surgically suctioning them from the body. The surgeon will make a small incision and use a cannula to vacuum loose fat deposits.

I strongly advise against liposuction as many women have reported adhesions, lumpiness from aggressive liposuction, internal scar tissue and unevenness in skin contours.

Conducting research for this book on realself.com only confirmed that liposuction is NOT the best cosmetic treatment option for cellulite.

The most common type of liposuction, tumescent liposuction, involves injecting medicated fluids into the area in which the fat will be removed in order to numb the tissues and reduce bleeding. The procedure is carried out under general anesthetic.

Pros: Liposuction is a good option for those looking to remove overall fat from an area, but it is not often recommended to solely treat cellulite. Liposuction can be very successful if combined with laser treatment (such as Cellulaze) and in the hands of a highly trained plastic surgeon.

Cons: Cellulite is made up of fat deposits near the surface of the skin. Liposuction generally targets fat that lies deeper in the body, and the effect on the appearance of cellulite **may be minimal.**

There is also the unfortunate possibility that your cellulite could end up looking even worse.

The price of liposuction can vary greatly depending on the surgeon and location, but on average, the procedure costs around $6000 to $10,000.

Chapter 8: Step-by-step Summary to Blast Cellulite

This final chapter is a summary of everything we have learned in the last six chapters about blasting cellulite.

This daily regime is by no means exhaustive – I have not included every possible treatment that this book discusses.

It's a sample workout routine and a weekly regime designed to smooth your cellulite, encourage collagen synthesis, and improve your circulation.

There are also two recipes for cellulite busting smoothies that you can use as a breakfast, snack, or post workout meal.

Day by day weekly regime

- Use coconut oil and start massaging your cellulite areas with the Fascia Blaster.
- On days that you are body brushing, dry brush before your shower and massage after to ensure optimal penetration of the cream into the skin.
- Do not complete the lower body workout more than three times a week.
- Feel free to add in your favorite cardio workouts throughout the

week, such as running, walking, cycling, or fitness classes.

Monday

- Kick Cellulite's Butt Lower Body Workout
- Fascia blast cellulite areas
- Apple Cinnamon Pie Smoothie

Tuesday

- Body brushing with dry brush
- Self-massage with cellulite cream

Wednesday

- Kick Cellulite's Butt Lower Body Workout
- Fascia blast cellulite areas
- Vitamin C Booster Smoothie

Thursday

- Body brushing with dry brush
- Self massage with cellulite cream

Friday

- Kick Cellulite's Butt Lower Body Workout
- Fascia blast cellulite areas
- Apple Cinnamon Pie Smoothie

Saturday

- Body brushing with dry brush
- Take a light walk

Sunday

- DIY slimming wrap
- Vitamin C Booster Smoothie

Cellulite Smoothing Smoothies

Vitamin C Booster Smoothie

Ingredients:

- 1 small banana
- ½ cup orange juice
- ½ cup low fat yogurt
- 5 strawberries
- 1 tbsp honey

Method:

- Blend all ingredients until smooth.
- Add more orange juice or water for a thinner consistency if you prefer.
- Keep for up to 12 hours in the refrigerator.

Apple Cinnamon Pie Smoothie

Ingredients:

- 1 small banana

- ¼ cup oats
- 1 tsp cinnamon
- 1 apple, peeled and chopped
- ½ cup milk
- ¼ cup apple juice
- ½ cup Greek yogurt

Method:

- Blend all ingredients until smooth. Add more orange juice or water for a thinner consistency if you prefer.
- Keep for up to 12 hours in the refrigerator.

Kick Cellulite's Butt Lower Body Workout

This workout is performed as a circuit. This means that you will move quickly from one exercise to the next with little rest in between. Use it on your cardio days, 3 times a week is sufficient.

This method of training increases cardiovascular activity and strengthens the muscles in an extremely time efficient manner.

- Do each exercise for 45 – 60 seconds before moving onto the next.
- Start by doing two circuits, and add more as your fitness increases.

- For further instruction on the exercises in this routine, refer to chapter 4.

Begin your workout with a five minute warm up. Choose your favorite pulse raising activity to warm your body before you engage in any workout routine.

Circuit 1
- Wall squat
- Barre raise
- Romanian dead lift
- Alternating reverse lunge
- Side step
- Sitting kick (right side)
- Bridge
- Inner thigh lift (left side)
- Donkey kick (left side)
- Fire hydrant (right side)

1 minute rest

Circuit 2

- Jumping squats
- Barre raise
- Romanian dead lift
- Jumping lunges
- Side step
- Sitting kick (left side)
- Bridge
- Inner thigh lift (right side)
- Donkey kick (right side)
- Fire hydrant (left side)

Cool down and stretch

Other Books By Aimee

HEALTH & BEAUTY SERIES

Book 1:

ACNE TREATMENT BOOK - The Adult Acne Treatment Book With Proven Acne Remedies & Treatments To Cure Cystic & Hormonal Acne For Radiant Skin

Book 2:

VOGUE HACKS - The 3 Step Intermittent Fasting System To Lose Up To 10 Pounds In 10 Days & Achieve Rapid Fat Loss.

Book 3:

10 YEARS YOUNGER - Look Younger With Yoga Face Exercises, Get Rid of Wrinkles & Take 10 Years off Your Face in 8 Mins A Day.

Book 4:

CELLULITE BLASTER - Quick Start Guide To Getting Rid Of Cellulite FAST and Blasting Them Off Your Stomach, Thighs, Legs & Butt!

You can find these books by "Aimee Blake" on the Amazon Kindle store at: **Amazon.com/author/aimeeblake**

About The Author

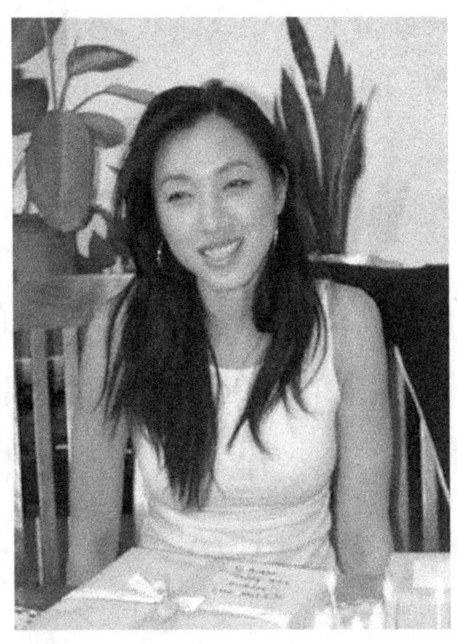

Aimee Blake is from Sydney Australia - she's a self experimenter of all things health, beauty and wellness and is a certified nutritionist.

In October 2013, she lost over 25 pounds in less than 2.5 months without restrictive diets, cardio whilst still eating the foods she loves!

This led her to writing "Vogue Hack" - a simple 3 step weight loss system that helps women with intermittent fasting, losing 10 pounds in 10 days and dropping a dress size fast!

She's written books on skin care and natural anti aging solutions and is committed to helping women all over the world improve their mind, body and spirit.

Thank You…And One Tiny Favor, Please

Thank you for reading my book! I really value your feedback and would appreciate it if you could leave a review.

As an independent author, I have a heart for helping people by sharing the information presented in this book.

Please leave me a helpful review on Amazon right now by turning to the last page.

It would really help benefit other people and zeus my doggy values your opinion as well!

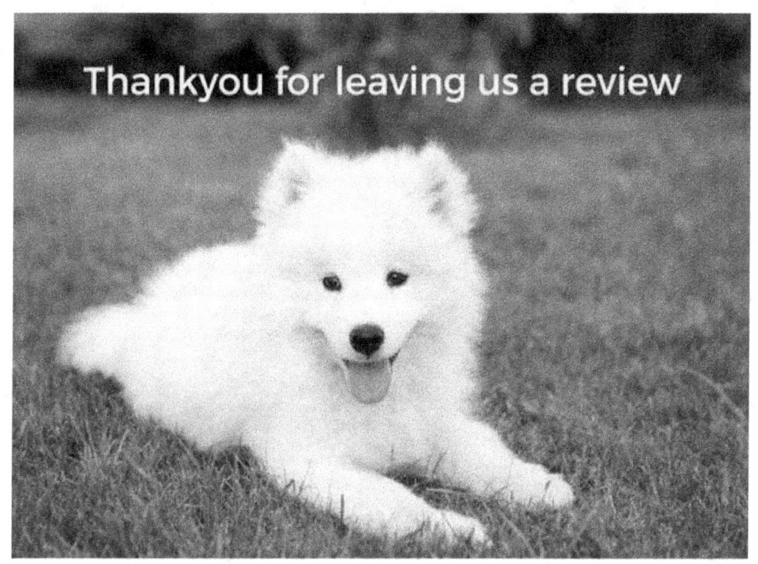
Thankyou for leaving us a review

www.ingramcontent.com/pod-product-compliance
Lightning Source LLC
Chambersburg PA
CBHW050927260726

48660CB00001B/434